Contents

INTRODUCTION

Oxalate is a naturally occurring molecule found in abundance in plants and humans. It's not a required nutrient for people, and too much can lead to kidney stones.

In plants, oxalate helps to get rid of extra calcium by binding with it. That is why so many high-oxalate foods are from plants.

When we eat foods with oxalate, it travels through the digestive tract and passes out in the stool or urine. As it passes through the intestines, oxalate can bind with calcium and be excreted in the stool. However, when too much oxalate continues through to the kidneys, it can lead to kidney stones.

Calcium oxalate kidney stones are the most common type of kidney stone in the U.S. The higher your levels of oxalate, the greater your risk of developing these kinds of kidney stones

If you are at high risk for kidney stones, lowering the amount of oxalate that you eat may help reduce this risk.

However, recent research indicates that boosting your intake of calcium-rich foods when you eat foods that are high in oxalate may be a better approach than simply eliminating it from the diet.

As they digest, oxalate and calcium are more likely to bind together before they get to the kidneys, making it less likely that kidney stones will form.

Foods that are high in vitamin C can increase the body's oxalate levels. Vitamin C converts to oxalate. Levels over 1,000 milligrams (mg) per day have been shown to increase oxalate levels.

Taking antibiotics, or having a history of digestive disease, can also increase the body's oxalate levels. The good bacteria in the gut help get rid of oxalate, and when the levels of these bacteria are low, higher amounts of oxalate can be absorbed in the body.

Drinking enough fluid each day can help clear kidney stones or even keep them from forming. Spreading your intake of liquids throughout the day is ideal. Choosing water over other drinks is preferable.

Avoid eating too much animal protein, as this can cause stones to form.

Getting enough calcium is also helpful. Getting too little calcium can increase the amount of oxalate that gets to the kidneys, which will increase the risk of kidney stones.

Lowering your salt intake can also lower your risk of kidney stones. High-salt diets tend to cause more calcium to be lost in the urine. The more calcium and oxalate in the kidneys, the greater the risk of kidney stones.

Many people are just learning of the benefits of limiting oxalates in their diet and are finding relief from symptoms such as inflammatory conditions, autoimmune issues, mineral deficiency, and perhaps even autism. Although chances are that you haven't heard of oxalate until now, odds are greater that you may have a form of oxalate intolerance or know someone suffering from symptoms of excess oxalate.

There is one way in which you can keep kidney stones at bay, and this involves reducing the number of oxalates that you consume. The other way you can reduce your chances of suffering kidney stones is by boosting your intake of calcium.

In this way, oxalates and calcium would bind before they got to the kidneys and this would prevent the formation of kidney stones. In the latter method, you would not have to reduce oxalates in your diet. However, studies show that reduction is the most suitable manner at the moment, as we await further advancements in the field.There is one way in which you can keep kidney stones at bay, and this involves reducing the number of oxalates that you consume. The other way you can reduce your chances of suffering kidney stones is by boosting your intake of calcium.

A low-carb diet is a diet that restricts carbohydrates, such as those found in sugary foods, pasta and bread. It is high in protein, fat and healthy vegetables.

This is a detailed meal plan for a low-carb diet. It explains what to eat, what to avoid and includes lot of low oxalate recipes!

CHAPTER ONE

What is Oxalic Acid?

Oxalic acid (ok-SAL-ik AS-id) is a transparent, colorless, crystalline solid that often occurs as the dihydrate (HOOCCOOH•2H2O). The dihydrate melts and begins to decompose at 101.5°C (214.7°F), forming the anhydrous acid. The compound is odorless, but has a characteristic tart, acidic taste. The acid should never be tasted, however, as it is very toxic.

Oxalic acid is one of the first organic acids to have been discovered and studied. It was first isolated by the German chemist Johann Christian Wiegleb (1732–1800) in 1769 and first synthesized by the Swedish chemist Karl Wilhelm Scheele (1742–1786) in 1776. Friedrich Wöhler's (1800–1882) synthesis of oxalic acid entirely from inorganic materials was a critical step in disproving the Vitalistic Theory of chemistry. The theory claimed that compounds found in living organisms could be produced only by the act of some supernatural being, and not by human actions.

HOW IT IS MADE

Traditionally, oxalic acid has been extracted from natural products by treating them with an alkaline solution, followed by crystallization of the acid. Sodium hydroxide is the alkaline material most commonly used for this procedure. Today, a number of methods are available for the commercial preparation of oxalic acid. In one procedure, carbon monoxide gas is bubbled through a concentrated solution of sodium hydroxide to produce oxalic acid. Alternatively, sodium formate (COONa) is heated in the presence of sodium hydroxide or sodium carbonate to obtain the acid. Another popular method of preparing oxalic acid involves the oxidation of sucrose (common table sugar) or more complex carbohydrates using nitric acid as a catalyst. The reaction results in the formation of oxalic acid and water as the primary products.

Biological Hazards:

Oxalic acid and oxalates are mild nephrotoxic acids that are abundantly present in many plants, most notably fat hen (lamb's quarters), rhubarb and sorrel. Oxalic acid irritates the lining of the gut when consumed, and can prove fatal in large doses. The LD50 for pure oxalic acid is predicted to be about 378 mg/kg body weight, or about 22 g for a 60 kg human. Oxalic acid can also be present in the body due to the consumption of another toxin, ethylene glycol (generally known as automobile antifreeze), because over time, the body metabolizes ethylene glycol partially into oxalic acid. Estimated fatal dose is 5 to 15 grams.

Bodily oxalic acid may also be synthesized via the metabolism of either glyoxylic acid or unused ascorbic acid (vitamin C), which is a serious health consideration for long term megadosers of vitamin C supplements. 80% of kidney stones are formed from calcium oxalate. Some Aspergillus species produce oxalic acid, which reacts with blood or tissue calcium to precipitate calcium oxalate. There is some preliminary evidence that the administration of probiotics can affect oxalic acid excretion rates (and presumably oxalic acid levels as well.)

Action of Poisoning:

Oxalic acid also combines with metals such as calcium, iron, sodium, magnesium, and potassium in the body to form oxalate crystals which precipitate and irritate the gut and kidneys. The calcium oxalate preciptate (better known as kidney stones) obstruct the kidney tubules. Because it binds vital nutrients such as calcium, long-term consumption of foods high in oxalic acid can lead to nutrient deficiencies.

Healthy individuals can safely consume such foods in moderation, but those with kidney disorders, gout, rheumatoid arthritis, or certain forms of chronic vulvar pain (vulvodynia) are typically advised to avoid foods high in oxalic acid or oxalates. Conversely, calcium supplements taken along with foods high in oxalic acid can cause oxalic acid to precipitate in the gut and drastically reduce the levels of oxalate absorbed by the body (by 97% in some cases.)

Symptoms of poisoning are weakness, burning in the mouth, death from cardiovascular collapse; on the respiratory system - difficulty breathing; on the eyes, ears, nose, and throat - burning in the throat; one the gastrointestinal system - abdominal pain, nausea, vomiting, diarrhea; and on the nervous system - Convulsions, coma.

What is oxalate?

Oxalate is a naturally occurring molecule found in abundance in plants and humans. It's not a required nutrient for people, and too much can lead to kidney stones.

In plants, oxalate helps to get rid of extra calcium by binding with it. That is why so many high-oxalate foods are from plants.

How does the body process it?

When we eat foods with oxalate, it travels through the digestive tract and passes out in the stool or urine. As it passes through the intestines, oxalate can bind with calcium and be excreted in the stool. However, when too much oxalate continues through to the kidneys, it can lead to kidney stones.

Calcium oxalate kidney stones are the most common type of kidney stone in the U.S. The higher your levels of oxalate, the greater your risk of developing these kinds of kidney stones.

What is a low-oxalate diet?

If you are at high risk for kidney stones, lowering the amount of oxalate that you eat may help reduce this risk.

However, recent research indicates that boosting your intake of calcium-rich foods when you eat foods that are high in oxalate may be a better approach than simply eliminating it from the diet.

As they digest, oxalate and calcium are more likely to bind together before they get to the kidneys, making it less likely that kidney stones will form.

What causes oxalate buildup?

Foods that are high in vitamin C can increase the body's oxalate levels. Vitamin C converts to oxalate. Levels over 1,000 milligrams (mg) per day have been shown to increase oxalate levels.

Taking antibiotics, or having a history of digestive disease, can also increase the body's oxalate levels. The good bacteria in the gut help get rid of oxalate, and when the levels of these bacteria are low, higher amounts of oxalate can be absorbed in the body.

What can reduce oxalate?

Drinking enough fluid each day can help clear kidney stones or even keep them from forming. Spreading your intake of liquids throughout the day is ideal. Choosing water over other drinks is preferable.

Avoid eating too much animal protein, as this can cause stones to form.

Getting enough calcium is also helpful. Getting too little calcium can increase the amount of oxalate that gets to the kidneys, which will increase the risk of kidney stones.

Lowering your salt intake can also lower your risk of kidney stones. High-salt diets tend to cause more calcium to be lost in the urine. The more calcium and oxalate in the kidneys, the greater the risk of kidney stones.

How is oxalate measured?

Lists that provide the oxalate content in foods can be confusing. The oxalate levels reported in foods can vary depending on the following factors:

• when the foods are harvested

• where they are grown

• how their oxalate levels were tested

Oxalate (Oxalic Acid): Good or Bad?

Leafy greens and other plant foods are very popular among the health-conscious.

However, many of these foods also contain an anti-nutrient called oxalate (oxalic acid).

Oxalic acid is an organic compound found in many plants.

These include leafy greens, vegetables, fruits, cocoa, nuts and seeds.

In plants, it's usually bound to minerals, forming oxalate. The terms "oxalic acid" and "oxalate" are used interchangeably in nutrition science.

Your body can produce oxalate on its own or obtain it from food. Vitamin C can also be converted into oxalate when it's metabolized.

Once consumed, oxalate can bind to minerals to form compounds, including calcium oxalate and iron oxalate. This mostly occurs in the colon, but can also take place in the kidneys and other parts of the urinary tract.

For most people, these compounds are then eliminated in the stool or urine.

However, for sensitive individuals, high-oxalate diets have been linked to an increased risk of kidney stones and other health problems.

BOTTOM LINE:

Oxalate is an organic acid found in plants, but can also be synthesized by the body. It binds minerals, and has been linked to kidney stones and other health problems.

Oxalate Can Reduce Mineral Absorption

One of the main health concerns about oxalate is that it can bind to minerals in the gut and prevent the body from absorbing them.

For example, spinach is high in calcium and oxalate, which prevents a lot of the calcium from being absorbed into the body.

Eating fiber and oxalate together may further hinder nutrient absorption.

Nevertheless, it's important to remember that only some of the minerals in our food will bind to oxalate.

Even though calcium absorption from spinach is reduced, calcium absorption from milk is not affected when milk and spinach are consumed together.

BOTTOM LINE:

Oxalate can bind to minerals in the gut and prevent some of them from being absorbed, particularly when combined with fiber.

Normally, calcium and small amounts of oxalate are present in the urinary tract at the same time, but they remain dissolved and cause no problems.

However, sometimes they bind to form crystals. In some people, these crystals can lead to the formation of stones, especially when oxalate is high and urine volume is low.

Small stones often don't cause any problems, but large stones can cause severe pain, nausea and blood in the urine as they move through the urinary tract.

Although there are other types of kidney stones, about 80% are made up of calcium oxalate.

For this reason, people who have had one episode of kidney stones may be advised to minimize their consumption of foods high in oxalate.

However, across-the-board oxalate restriction is no longer recommended to every person with kidney stones. This is because most of the oxalate found in urine is produced by the body, rather than absorbed from food.

Most urologists now only prescribe a strict low-oxalate diet (less than 50 milligrams per day) for patients who have high levels of oxalate in their urine.

Therefore, it's important to be tested from time to time to figure out how much restriction is necessary.

BOTTOM LINE:

High-oxalate foods may increase the risk of kidney stones in susceptible people, and recommendations for patients are based on urinary levels.

Some claim that a high oxalate intake may be linked to the development of autism.

Others say oxalates may be linked to vulvodynia, which is characterized by chronic, unexplained vaginal pain.

Based on study results, researchers believe neither of these disorders are likely triggered by dietary oxalates.

However, when 59 women with vulvodynia were treated with a low-oxalate diet and calcium supplements, nearly a quarter experienced improvements in symptoms.

The authors of that study concluded that dietary oxalate might worsen, rather than cause, the condition.

Several online anecdotes do link oxalates with autism and vulvodynia, but only a few studies have looked into possible connections. Further research is needed.

BOTTOM LINE:

Some people have suggested that consuming foods high in oxalate may lead to autism and vulvodynia, but at this point the research does not support these claims.

Most Foods with Oxalates Are Very Healthy

Some proponents of low-oxalate diets say people are better off not consuming foods rich in oxalates, since they may have negative health effects.

However, it's not that simple. Many of these are healthy foods that contain important antioxidants, fiber and other nutrients.

Therefore, it's not a good idea for most people to completely stop eating high-oxalate foods.

BOTTOM LINE:

Many foods that contain oxalates are delicious and provide many health benefits. Avoiding them is not necessary for most people, and may even be detrimental

Your Gut Determines Oxalate Absorption

Some of the oxalate you eat can be broken down by bacteria in the gut, which happens before it can bind to minerals.

One of them, Oxalobacter formigenes, actually uses it as an energy source. It significantly reduces the amount your body absorbs.

However, some people don't have much of this bacteria in their gut, as antibiotics decrease the number of O. formigenes colonies.

What's more, studies have found that people with inflammatory bowel disease have an increased risk of developing kidney stones.

This is partly because they are unable to regulate the amount of oxalate they absorb.

Similarly, elevated levels of oxalate have been found in the urine of patients who have had gastric bypass surgery or other surgeries that alter gut function.

This suggests that people who have taken antibiotics or suffer from gut dysfunction may benefit more from a low-oxalate diet.

BOTTOM LINE:

Most healthy people can consume oxalate-rich foods without problems, but those with altered gut function may need to limit their intake.

Why are there crystals in my urine?

Urine contains a large number of different chemicals. Under some circumstances, these chemicals may solidify into salt crystals. This is called crystalluria.

Crystals can be found in the urine of healthy individuals. They may be caused by minor issues like a slight excess of protein or vitamin C. Many types of urine crystals are relatively harmless.

In some cases, however, urine crystals can be indicators of a more serious underlying condition. Symptoms that would indicate a more serious condition could include:

• fever

• severe abdominal pain

• blood in the urine

• jaundice

• fatigue

Types of urine crystals

There are a number of different types of urine crystals.

Uric acid

Uric acid crystals can be different types of shapes: barrel, plate-like, or diamond. They're typically orange-brown or yellow in color.

They can be found in normal urine when caused by a protein-rich diet, which increases uric acid in the urine.

They can also be caused by kidney stones, gout, chemotherapy, or tumor lysis syndrome.

Symptoms of kidney stones include severe abdominal, flank, or groin pain; nausea; and blood in the urine. Symptoms of gout can include burning pain, stiffness, and swelling in a joint.

Treatment depends on the underlying condition, but staying hydrated is one of the best ways to treat the crystals themselves.

Calcium oxalate

Calcium oxalate crystals are shaped like dumbbells or envelopes. They're colorless and can be found in healthy urine.

Calcium oxalate crystals are heavily associated with kidney stones, which can form when too much oxalate (found in such foods as spinach) is in the system. Kidney stone symptoms include severe groin or abdominal pain, nausea, fever, and difficulty passing urine. These natural remedies can help you fight kidney stones at home.

In some cases, calcium oxalate crystals can be caused by the ingestion of ethylene glycol, which is toxic and is an essential ingredient in antifreeze formulations. Exposure to this compound can cause symptoms such as:

• throat and lung irritation

• central nervous system problems

• renal failure

Your doctor may recommend dietary changes to reduce oxalate in your diet and increase hydration. They'll also likely recommend that you reduce salty foods.

Hippuric

Hippuric acid crystals are rare. They may be either yellow-brown or clear, and they often resemble needle-like prisms or plates. Hippuric acid crystals are often found clustered together.

While they are sometimes caused by an acidic urine pH, hippuric acid crystals can also occur in healthy urine.

Magnesium ammonium phosphate (struvite)

Magnesium ammonium phosphate crystals are often colorless, rectangular prisms. They can be found in healthy urine, but they typically coincide with a urinary tract infection (UTI). Other symptoms of UTIs include:

• cloudy urine

• frequent, intense urge to urinate

• chills

• nausea

• fatigue

• lower back pain

• fever

If a UTI is causing these crystals, your doctor will prescribe you antibiotics to clear up the infection.

Calcium carbonate

Calcium carbonate crystals are large, round discs with smooth surfaces. They're often a light brown color. Crystals of calcium carbonate — which is a supplement you can take to get more calcium — are also frequently associated with kidney stones.

If you have calcium carbonate crystals in your urine, your doctor may recommend obtaining calcium through other means, like adding more dairy to your diet, instead of supplements.

Bilirubin is made when the healthy destruction of red blood cells occurs. It's passed through the liver.

Bilirubin crystals have a needle-like, granular appearance and are often very small and yellow in color. High levels of bilirubin or bilirubin crystals in your urine could indicate liver disease or poor liver function. Other symptoms may include nausea, pain, vomiting, jaundice, and fever.

Treatment depends on the underlying cause. Medications may be used to change the amount of protein that's absorbed in the diet, especially in cases of cirrhosis.

Calcium phosphate

Calcium phosphate crystals are colorless and may appear as star-like or needle-like, though they may also form plates. They may show up alone or in clusters. They often appear in alkaline urine, though they can be found in normal urine.

In rare cases, calcium phosphate crystals could by caused by hypoparathyroidism. Symptoms of this include tingling in the hands and muscle cramping.

Treatment may include drinking more water, getting more calcium, and taking vitamin D supplements.

These crystals are brown spheres with spiky thorns. They almost resemble small bugs. They're often found in alkaline urine, but they can also be seen in normal urine.

Sometimes ammonium biurate crystals only appear because the urine sample is old or has been poorly preserved. Because of this, recollecting a urine sample may be advised if these crystals appear.

Cholesterol

Cholesterol crystals are often clear and shaped like long rectangles, with a notch cut out at the corner. They're most likely to appear after a urine sample has been refrigerated.

Cholesterol crystals can be found in both neutral and acid urine. They may be caused by renal tubular disease, which can lead to renal failure if left untreated.

Treatment may involve alkali therapy to help treat chronic metabolic conditions, like renal tubular disease.

Cystine

Cystine is an amino acid, and it can cause urine crystals and kidney stones. Kidney stones caused by cystine acid are typically larger than most other kidney stones. It's a rare condition, and often genetic.

The condition that causes cystine to bind together and form the crystals is called cystinuria. The crystals, when found in urine, are often shaped like hexagons and may be colorless. Symptoms may include blood in the urine, nausea and vomiting, and pain in the groin or back.

Your doctor may prescribe chelating medications, which help to dissolve the crystals.

Leucine

These crystals are yellow-brown discs with concentric rings like a tree trunk. Leucine crystals typically aren't found in healthy urine. They're found in acidic urine. They're usually a symptom of severe liver disease. Other symptoms may include abdominal swelling, vomiting, nausea, disorientation, and malaise.

Treatment involves improving liver function and health immediately. This will include medications to reduce the risk of bleeding and reduce swelling caused by excess fluid.

Tyrosine

Tyrosine crystals are colorless and needle-like. They're often found in acidic urine, and they may be caused by metabolic disorders like liver disease or tyrosinemia. Symptoms of tyrosinemia include difficulty gaining weight, fever, diarrhea, bloody stools, and vomiting.

Treatment includes exercising, eating a healthy diet, and taking medications that may be able to treat high blood pressure, high cholesterol, and diabetes.

Indinavir

Indinavir is a medication used to treat HIV. It can cause the formation of crystals in the urine. Indinavir crystals may resemble starbursts, rectangular plates, or fans. Other symptoms of indinavir crystals may include back or flank pain.

How are urine crystals diagnosed?

If your doctor suspects that you have urine crystals, they'll likely first order a urinalysis. In some cases, your doctor may run a urinalysis as part of your wellness visit or annual checkup, even if you don't have other complaints.

For the urinalysis test, you'll be asked to provide a urine sample. The lab technician reviewing the sample will first observe it for any color or cloudiness that may indicate an infection. Bilirubin can turn urine a dark tea color, for example. Blood may be evident to the naked eye.

They'll then use a dipstick to test for components within the urine.

The technician will finally examine the sample under a microscope, where they can actually see the crystals if any have formed.

Depending on what your doctor finds, they may order additional tests. If they find bilirubin in your urine, for example, they may order blood work or an ultrasound to evaluate your liver health. If urine crystals indicate high cholesterol, they'll order a blood test to evaluate your current cholesterol levels.

Is this preventable?

Urine crystals that aren't caused by underlying conditions like liver disease or genetic conditions can often be prevented. In some cases, even crystalluria triggered by genetic causes can be reduced with lifestyle or diet changes.

The most effective way to prevent urine crystals is to drink more water and stay hydrated. This helps dilute the chemical concentrations in the urine, preventing crystals from forming.

You can also make certain changes in your diet. Your doctor can help you determine what changes to make based on the type of crystals that you have. They may recommend cutting back on protein, for example, or reducing foods high in oxalate (as is the case for calcium oxalate crystals).

Avoiding salty foods can also help prevent a number of different urine crystals, so eliminating processed foods can be beneficial.

What's the outlook?

In many instances, urine crystals are highly treatable with lifestyle and diet changes. In some cases, medication may be required to treat underlying conditions.

If you experience any changes in your urine, make an appointment to see your doctor. Knowing exactly what type of crystals are forming will help you and your doctor to understand what's causing the issue and how to treat it.

What are calcium oxalate crystals?

Calcium oxalate crystals are the most common cause of kidney stones — hard clumps of minerals and other substances that form in the kidneys. These crystals are made from oxalate — a substance found in foods like green, leafy vegetables — combined with calcium. Having too much oxalate or too little urine can cause the oxalate to crystalize and clump together into stones.

Kidney stones can be very painful. They can also cause complications like urinary tract infections. But they are often preventable with a few dietary changes.

Where does oxalate come from?
Oxalate comes from many of the foods in our diet. The main dietary sources of oxalate are:

• spinach and other green, leafy vegetables

• rhubarb

• wheat bran

• almonds

• beets

• navy beans

• chocolate

• okra

• French fries and baked potatoes

• nuts and seeds

• soy products

• tea

• strawberries and raspberries

When you eat these foods, your GI tract breaks them down and absorbs the nutrients. The leftover wastes then travel to your kidneys, which remove them into your urine. The waste from broken-down oxalate is called oxalic acid. It can combine with calcium to form calcium oxalate crystals in the urine.

What are the symptoms?

Kidney stones may not cause symptoms until they start to move through your urinary tract. When stones move, the pain can be intense.

The main symptoms of calcium oxalate crystals in the urine are:

• pain in your side and back that can be intense, and may come in waves

• pain when you urinate

• blood in your urine, which can look red, pink, or brown

• cloudy urine

• foul-smelling urine

• an urgent and constant need to urinate

• nausea and vomiting

• fever and chills if you have an infection

What causes calcium oxalate crystals?

Urine contains chemicals that normally prevent oxalate from sticking together and forming crystals. However, if you have too little urine or too much oxalate, it can crystalize and form stones. Reasons for this include:

• not drinking enough fluids (being dehydrated)

• eating a diet that's too high in oxalate, protein, or salt

In other cases, an underlying disease causes the crystals to form into stones. You're more likely to get calcium oxalate stones if you have:

• hyperparathyroidism, or too much parathyroid hormone

• inflammatory bowel disease (IBD), such as ulcerative colitis or Crohn's disease

• Dent disease, an inherited disorder that damages the kidneys

• gastric bypass surgery for weight loss

• diabetes

• obesity

How are they diagnosed?

Your doctor might use these tests to find out if you have calcium oxalate stones:

Urine test. Your doctor may request a 24-hour urine sample to check levels of oxalate in your urine. You'll have to collect your urine throughout the day for 24 hours. A normal urine oxalate level is less than 45 milligrams (mg) per day.

Blood test. Your doctor can test your blood for the gene mutation that causes Dent disease.

Imaging tests. An X-ray or CT scan can show stones in your kidney.

What happens during pregnancy?

During pregnancy, blood flow increases to nourish your growing baby. More blood gets filtered through your kidneys, which causes more oxalate to be removed into your urine. Even though the risk of kidney stones is the same during pregnancy as it is during other times of your life, extra oxalate in your urine can promote stone formation.

Kidney stones can cause complications during pregnancy. Some studies have shown that stones increase the risks for miscarriage, preeclampsia, gestational diabetes, and a cesarean delivery.

During pregnancy, imaging tests like a CT scan or X-ray may not be safe for your baby. Your doctor can use an ultrasound to diagnose you instead.

Up to 84 percent of stones pass on their own during pregnancy. About half of the stones that don't pass during pregnancy will pass after delivery.

If you're having severe symptoms from the kidney stone, or your pregnancy is at risk, procedures like a stent or lithotripsy can remove the stone.

What's the treatment?

Small stones may pass on their own without treatment in about four to six weeks. You can help flush out the stone by drinking extra water.

Your doctor can also prescribe an alpha-blocker like doxazosin (Cardura) or tamsulosin (Flomax). These drugs relax your ureter to help the stone pass from your kidney more quickly.

Pain relievers such as ibuprofen (Advil, Motrin) and acetaminophen (Tylenol) can help relieve your discomfort until the stone passes. However, if you're pregnant, talk with your healthcare provider before taking non-steroidal, anti-inflammatory drugs (ibuprofen, naproxen, aspirin, and celexcoxib).

If the stone is very large or it doesn't pass on its own, you may need one of these procedures to remove it:

Extracorporeal shock wave lithotripsy (ESWL). ESWL delivers sound waves from outside your body to break the stone into little pieces. Within a few weeks after ESWL, you should pass the stone pieces in your urine.

Ureteroscopy. In this procedure, your doctor passes a thin scope with a camera on the end through your bladder and into your kidney. Then the stone is either removed in a basket or broken up first with a laser or other tools and then removed. The surgeon may place a thin plastic tube called a stent in the ureter to hold it open and allow urine to drain while you heal.

Percutaneous nephrolithotomy. This procedure occurs while you're asleep and pain-free under general anesthesia. Your surgeon makes a small incision in your back and removes the stone using small instruments.

How can you prevent calcium oxalate crystals?

You can prevent calcium oxalate from forming crystals in your urine and avoid kidney stones by following these tips:

• Drink extra fluids. Some doctors recommend that people who've had kidney stones drink 2.6 quarts (2.5 liters) of water each day. Ask your doctor how much fluid is right for you.

• Limit the salt in your diet. A high-sodium diet can increase the amount of calcium in your urine, which can help stones form.

• Watch your protein intake. Protein is essential to a healthy diet, but don't overdo it. Too much of this nutrient can cause stones to form. Make protein less than 30 percent of your total daily calories.

• Include the right amount of calcium in your diet. Getting too little calcium in your diet can cause oxalate levels to rise. To prevent this, be sure you're getting the appropriate daily amount of calcium for your age. Ideally, you'll want to get calcium from foods like milk and cheese. Some studies have linked calcium supplements (when not taken with a meal) to kidney stones.

• Cut down on foods that are high in oxalate, like rhubarb, bran, soy, beets, and nuts. When you do eat oxalate-rich foods, have them with something containing calcium, like a glass of milk. This way the oxalate will bind to calcium before it gets to your kidneys, so it won't crystallize in your urine. Learn more about a low-oxalate diet.

If you've had calcium oxalate stones in the past, or you have symptoms of stones, see your primary care doctor or a urologist. Find out what changes you should make to your diet to prevent these stones from forming again.

What foods should I include?

Include the following foods that have a low to medium amount of oxalate.

Grains:

• Egg noodles

• Graham crackers

• Pancakes and waffles

• Cooked and dry cereals without nuts or bran

• White or wild rice

• White bread, cornbread, bagels, and white English muffins (medium oxalate)

• Saltine or soda crackers and vanilla wafers (medium oxalate)

• Brown rice, spaghetti, and other noodles and pastas (medium oxalate)

Fruit:

• Apples, bananas, grapes

• Grapefruit and cranberries

• Peaches, nectarines, apricots, and pears

• Papayas and strawberries

• Melons and pineapples

• Blackberries, blueberries, mangoes, and prunes (medium oxalate)

Vegetables:

• Artichokes, asparagus, and brussels sprouts

• Broccoli and cauliflower

• Kale, endive, cabbage, and lettuce

• Cucumbers, peas, and zucchini

• Mushrooms, onions, and peppers

• Potatoes and corn

• Carrots, celery, and green beans (medium oxalate)

• Parsnips, summer squash, tomatoes, and turnips (medium oxalate)

Dairy:

• American cheese, Swiss cheese, cottage cheese, ricotta cheese, and cheddar cheese

- Milk and buttermilk

- Yogurt

Protein foods:

- Meat, fish, shellfish, chicken, and turkey

- Lunch meat and ham (medium oxalate)

- Hot dogs, bratwurst, bacon, and sausage (medium oxalate)

Drinks and desserts:

- Coffee

- Fruit punch and lemonade or limeade without added vitamin C

Desserts:

- Cookies, cakes, and ice cream

- Pudding without chocolate

What foods should I limit or avoid?

Limit the following foods that are high in oxalate.

Grains:

- Wheat bran, wheat germ, and barley

- Grits and bran cereal

- White corn flour and buckwheat flour

- Whole wheat bread

Fruit:

• Dried apricots

• Red currants, figs, and rhubarb

• Kiwi

Vegetables:

• Collard greens, leeks, okra, and spinach

• Wax beans

• Eggplant

• Beets and beet greens

• Swiss chard, escarole, parsley, and rutabagas

• Tomato paste

Protein foods:

• Baked beans with tomato sauce

• Nut butters and nuts (peanuts, almonds, pecans, cashews, hazelnuts)

• Soy burgers

• Miso

• Dried bean

Desserts:

• Fruitcake

• Chocolate

• Carob and marmalade

Beverages:

• Chocolate drink mixes

• Soy milk

• Instant iced tea

Other foods:

• Sesame seeds and tahini (paste made of sesame seeds)

• Poppy seeds

What other dietary guidelines should I follow?

Drink about 12 to 16 (eight-ounce) cups of liquid each day. Liquids help clear kidney stones and prevent them from forming again. Water is the best liquid to drink. You may need more liquid if you are physically active. Ask your healthcare provider or dietitian how much liquid you need to drink each day.

Your healthcare provider may suggest that you make other diet changes to help prevent kidney stones. This may include decreasing the amount of sodium you eat each day.

High-calcium foods

Increasing your calcium intake when eating foods with oxalate can help lower oxalate levels in the urine. Choose high-calcium dairy foods such as milk, yogurt, and cheese.

Vegetables can also provide a good amount of calcium. Choose among the following foods to increase your calcium levels:

• broccoli

• watercress

• kale

• okra

High-calcium legumes that have a fair amount of calcium include:

• kidney beans

• chickpeas

• baked beans

• navy beans

Fish with a lot of calcium include:

• sardines with bones

• whitebait

• salmon

How to Do a Low-Oxalate Diet

People who are placed on low-oxalate diets for kidney stones are usually instructed to eat less than 50 mg of it each day.

Here are a few tips on how to follow a low-oxalate diet:

• Limit oxalate to 50 mg per day: Choose a variety of nutrient-dense animal and plant sources from this list of foods very low in oxalate.

• Boil oxalate-rich vegetables: Boiling vegetables can reduce their oxalate content from 30% to almost 90%, depending on the vegetable.

• Drink plenty of water: Aim for a minimum of 2 liters daily. If you have kidney stones, drink enough to produce at least 2.5 liters of urine a day.

• Get enough calcium: Calcium binds to oxalate in the gut and reduces the amount your body absorbs, so try to get about 800–1,200 mg per day.

Foods high in calcium and low in oxalate include:

• Cheese

• Plain yogurt

• Canned fish with bones

• Bok choy

• Broccoli

BOTTOM LINE:

Diets with less than 50 mg of oxalate per day can be balanced and nutritious. Calcium also helps reduce its absorption.

Should You Avoid it?

People who tend to form kidney stones may benefit from a low-oxalate diet.

However, healthy people trying to stay healthy do NOT need to avoid nutrient-dense foods just because they are high in oxalates.

It is simply not a nutrient of concern for most people.

Recipes

COCONUT FLOUR CHOCOLATE CHIP COOKIES

So easy to make, bake and enjoy! Use coconut flour and coconut oil to make these delicious cookies.

Course   Dessert

Cuisine   American

Prep Time   20 minutes

Cook Time   20 minutes

Total Time   40 minutes

Author   The Savvy Age

Ingredients:

1/3 cup coconut flour

1/4 cup coconut oil melted

1/4 cup maple syrup

1 tsp. vanilla extract

1/4 tsp. salt

2 whole eggs

1/3 cup dark chocolate or semi sweet chips

Instructions:

Preheat oven to 350 degrees.

Line a baking sheet with parchment paper or parchment paper sheets.

In a medium size bowl, combine coconut flour, melted and cooled coconut oil, syrup, eggs vanilla and salt.

Whisk mixture together.

Allow dough to sit five minutes so the dough thickens.

Add the chocolate chips.

Using a tablespoon or cookie scoop, drop 12 cookies onto baking sheet.

Bake 13-14 minutes and remove from oven when the edges begin to turn golden brown.

Cool.

Notes: Store cookies in refrigerator.

Rainbow Cauliflower White Pizza

Choose your favorite vegetable toppings, white cheese and a cauliflower pizza crust to make bake a homemade and healthy white pizza (rainbow design optional!) aka Rainbow Cauliflower White Pizza recipe.

Course   Main Course

Cuisine   American

Keyword   cauliflower white pizza

Prep Time   10 minutes

Cook Time   10 minutes

Total Time   20 minutes

Servings 4

Ingredients:

Favorite Cauliflower pizza crust

Ricotta Cheese

Favorite Veggies or favorite low oxalate vegetables

Instructions:

Bake your cauliflower pizza crisp according to the directions.

Chop and dice the vegetables.

When the pizza crust is 75% baked I remove the pizza crust from the oven and spread a healthy layer of ricotta on top of the crust.

Return pizza crust to oven to warm and melt the cheese.

Once the cheese is melted and warmed I add the vegetables.

Butternut Squash Bake With Apples

Easy to make and a healthy side dish using butternut squash and apples. Fluffy "bake" combines the best of butternut squash and apples (or applesauce) for a versatile side dish which can also be a dessert!

Course Side Dish

Cuisine American

Keyword butternut squash apple bake

Prep Time 20 minutes

Cook Time 30 minutes

Total Time 50 minutes

Servings: 8

Ingredients:

1 10 ounce bag of frozen butternut squash OR 1 medium butternut squash about 1.5 pounds works well

1 tablespoon butter

1/2 teaspoon salt

1/4 teaspoon pepper

3 medium apples peeled and cored *** or 12 oz. applesauce

1/4 teaspoon cinnamon

1 tablespoon sugar

Need to add some crunch to the ? This is a very flexible and very forgiving side dish. A crunchy sweet topping can be added to the entire dish or just half the dish to satisfy all ! Add the topping before baking.

Topping:

1 cup slightly crushed cornflakes

1/4 cup chopped pecans or the nut of your choice

1 tablespoon melted butter

1 tablespoon brown sugar

Mix into a crumble and add to the Butternut Squash Apple Bake before baking.

Or skip the crumble and just add your favorite nuts to the top after baking.

Instructions:

Preheat oven to 350 degrees.

Microwave the butternut squash per directions on the bag. If using fresh butternut squash peel squash, remove seeds, cut into large pieces. This is the most labor intensive part of the recipe, it

can be tough to tame a butternut squash, be careful! Boil squash for 20-30 minutes until tender. Drain.

In a medium bowl, add the butternut squash and very gently mash a few of the pieces.

Add remaining ingredients and gently mix. This will determine the smoothness of the dish.

Spoon into a 9" pie dish or an 8" square glass dish. The consistency will be fluffy!

Bake 25-30 minutes at 350 degrees.

Need to add some crunch to the ? This is a very flexible and very forgiving side dish. A crunchy sweet topping can be added to the entire dish or just half the dish to satisfy all ! Add the topping before baking.

Copycat PF Chang's Lettuce Wrap Recipe

Great way to use leftover chicken! Copycat PF Chang's Lettuce Wraps recipe is a close match to the original and low oxalate too!

Course Main Course

Cuisine American, Chinese

Keyword Copycat PF Chang's Lettuce Wraps recipe

Prep Time 15 minutes

Cook Time 5 minutes

Total Time 20 minutes

Servings 4

Ingredients:

1-1.5 breasts of leftover seasoned chicken or rotisserie chicken depends upon size of chicken breast

1 can of water chestnuts

2 tablespoons low sodium soy sauce

2 tablespoons of brown sugar sugar substitute if watching sugar intake

1/2 teaspoon rice vinegar

1 teaspoon minced garlic

2 to 3 tablespoons dried chives or fresh chives

1 tablespoon of cooking oil or olive for stir fry

Iceberg lettuce or white rice or rice sticks

Instructions:

Chop the water chestnuts and chicken into dice size pieces.

Mix together: low sodium soy sauce sauce, brown sugar, garlic, chives and rice vinegar.

Heat one tablespoon of oil in a large frying pan at medium high heat.

Add the diced chicken and water chestnuts to the pan and then add the stir fry sauce. Cook for five five minutes on medium heat then lower to medium low heat for an additional three to five minutes.

Ready to serve! Use leaves of iceberg lettuce as the wrap for the traditional recipe or serve over white rice. Rice Sticks are optional for oxalate friendly guests; however rice flour which is the main ingredient in rice sticks are high on the oxalate list.

Simply gather your fresh gluten-free ingredients and you are ready to assemble this crispy flavorful snack. Sweet banana combines with the kick of apple butter and the crispy cereal coating for bite size treats perfect for breakfast or a snack anytime of the day.

INGREDIENTS APPLE BANANA SUSHI:

• Banana

• Gluten-Free Apple Butter

• Gluten-Free Krispy Cereal (brand of your choice)

Directions:

• Peel the banana

• Spread apple butter on the outside of banana

• Spread the cereal on a paper plate

• Roll banana in the cereal mixture

• Cut the finished sushi into bite size slices

Kitchen Tip: If you are using a newly purchased jar of gluten-free apple butter, chilling the apple butter makes spreading the apple butter on the banana much easier!

Low Oxalate Ham Broccoli Crustless Quiche

Light and airy low oxalate ham and broccoli crustless quiche the whole family can enjoy!

Course Main Course

Cuisine American

Keyword low oxalate ham and broccoli crustless quiche

Prep Time 15 minutes

Cook Time 30 minutes

Total Time 45 minutes

Servings 4

Ingredients:

1 cup diced ham can use low salt ham

1 cup broccoli florets frozen or fresh

4 eggs

4 egg whites

1/4 cup water

1 cup low fat cottage cheese

White pepper to taste

Instructions:

Prepare a 9 " pie, baking dish or quiche dish with cooking spray.

Heat oven to 375 degrees.

Prepare your broccoli by pre cooking either in the microwave or on the stove top.

Dice the ham while the broccoli is cooking.

Using a large bowl, whisk the eggs, egg whites and water.

Now add the cottage cheese and whisk with intent! You want the cottage cheese to become fairly smooth and mix in with the egg mixture.

Pour into prepared dish. Place the broccoli and ham into the mixture.

Bake for 30 to 35 minutes. Check at the 30 minute mark.

As there is no crust, the top of the Ham And Broccoli Crustless Quiche will be slightly brown and the edges will be sightly brown also.

Enjoy this easy No Bake Watermelon Cake recipe! The healthy cake perfect for picnics, barbecues and birthday parties.

Course Dessert

Cuisine American

Keyword watermelon cake

Prep Time 20 minutes

Servings 4

Ingredients:

Watermelon whole or half or round. Seedless preferred.

Fresh berries or fruit of your choice for decoration.

Whipped cream for frosting Coconut for Paleo friendly

Nuts decorating sprinkles if desired

Instructions:

"Baking" The Watermelon Cake

Cut your watermelon into the desired shape.

I began with a small round seedless watermelon and cut the watermelon into a rectangle. For obvious reasons, a seedless watermelon does promote friendly consumption.

Frost with your choice of store purchased or homemade whipped cream. I have tried this cake with the canned whipped cream and homemade whipped cream or coconut frosting.

The taste of the homemade whipped cream was superior; however, for ease and consistency, the canned whipped cream was easier to apply.

Frosting The Watermelon Cake:

After choosing the frosting (a coconut milk based whipped cream is also a good choice) frost the watermelon cake just as any other cake.

If you are making your own whipped cream please remember a thicker consistency is desired as it adheres better to the watermelon and allows for easier decoration.

Feel free to use the whipped cream frosting of your choice. There is a little trial and error involved to perfect the consistency which will adhere to the cake.

It will be apparent very quickly if your frosting needs to be thickened a smidge to adhere to the watermelon cake.

There are quite a few recipes for coconut frosting listed at Allrecipes if you are interested in trying a coconut frosting. I find the reviews invaluable for tips and tweaking of a recipe.

Chill until serving.

LOW OXALATE HELLO DOLLY BAR

Chances are if you've landed here then you are familiar with low oxalates and the medical conditions which suggest the benefit of a low oxalate meal plan. As always medical professionals should advise as to your dietary requirements. Perhaps you've been given "the" low oxalate list and as oxalate researchers discover there is not one list, lists contradict each other regarding which foods are low oxalate and the value of oxalates in the same food. But enough of that! (I suspect you've already discovered that.)

Ingredients:

1.5 cups corn flake crumbs

1/2 cup unsalted butter

1 cup white chocolate chips

1 cup butterscotch chips

1 cup chopped macadamia nuts

1 1/3 cups shredded coconut

1 14 oz. can sweetened condensed milk

Directions:

Heat oven to 350 degrees.

Line a 13 X 9 baking pan with parchment paper. The entire pan should be lined.

Cut up butter, place in baking pan and put in oven until butter is melted.

Melt butter in the microwave. Add cornflake crumbs to butter and lightly mix. Add mixture to parchment lined pan and lightly press the mixture into a cornflake crumb layer.

Sprinkle chopped nuts over the cornflake crumb layer.

Sprinkle semi sweet chocolate chips over the cornflake crumb layer.

Sprinkle butterscotch chips over the cornflake crumb layer.

Pour condensed milk over mixture.

Sprinkle coconut over top of bars.

Cook at 350 degrees for 25 minutes. The coconut should be very lightly browned.

Cool. Using the parchment paper as handles lift the Low Oxalate Hello Dolly Bars out of the baking pan.

Cut into squares.

Nuts Not Necessary!

I have included macadamia nuts in this recipe as they are one of the lowest oxalate nuts and the quantity is low in relation to chopped nuts spread over a 13 X 9 pan. However nuts can also be eliminated for this recipe. I have made the dessert bars without nuts and the taste difference is negligibly.

Sweet And Salty Puffcorn

No Bake Puffcorn recipe for the ultimate sweet and salty party snack.

Course: Snack

Cuisine: American

Keyword: Sweet and salty puffcorn

Prep Time: 15 minutes

Total Time: 15 minutes

Servings: 8

Ingredients:

1 bag of Puffcorn Chesters brand is my favorite

1/2 bar of almond bark or 1/2 bag of white chocolate chips

2 cookie sheets

Parchment paper

Sprinkles jimmies, edible decorations

Instructions:

Line 2 cookie sheets with parchment paper. Wax paper will also work.

Spread the puffcorn in a single layer on two cookie sheets.

Melt the bark or white chocolate chips in a microwave safe bowl. I begin by melting the chocolate/bark in 30 second increments.

With a wooden spoon drizzle the chocolate onto the puffcorn. The amount of drizzle is up to you. It is okay to be generous, the majority of the puffcorn should have a 'touch' of chocolate drizzle.

If desired, decorate the puffcorn with sprinkles, jimmies or any edible decoration.

Set the puffcorn on the counter for approximately 15 minutes. For a quick set pop the cookie sheets into the refrigerator.

Break apart the puffcorn into finger food size morsels.

Store in an airtight container.

Notes

Puffcorn also known as hullless popcorn is in the snack aisle of grocery stores and convenience stores. The major brands of puffcorn include Chesters (by Frito Lay), Bettermade, Herr, Meijer. The puffcorn can be plain or butter flavored.

Halloween Popcorn Ball Lollipops

This was a blast from Halloween's of the past to make Halloween Popcorn Ball Lollipops! Easy Halloween treat for kids and adults too!

Course Dessert

Cuisine American

Keyword Easy Halloween food Idea, Halloween Popcorn Ball Lollipops

Prep Time 30 minutes

Set time 15 minutes

Total Time 45 minutes

Servings 24 Lollipops

Ingredients:

10 ounces miniature marshmallows

8 cups of popped popcorn

1/4 cup butter

Optional: 1 teaspoon extract vanilla or almond extract

Lollipop Sticks pack of 100

Lots of Halloween sprinkles

Orange food coloring if making Orange Lollipops

Candy eyeballs

Candy Corn optional

Instructions:

This is a very quick and very easy recipe. No muss, no fuss!

In a medium pan under low heat, add the marshmallows and butter.

Stir continuously until the butter and marshmallows melt.

Remove from heat.

Stir in popcorn. (Sticky alert!) I coat my wooden spoon with cooking spray to help stir the popcorn in the marshmallow mixture.

Now the fun part! Mix in your desired amount of Halloween sprinkles.

I use the sprinkle, mix, evaluate method before just dumping in a bunch of sprinkles, but the dump and stir method works too. For little kids to participate the dump and stir method works very well!

Using disposable gloves I spritz cooking spray on the gloves to help form the popcorn ball lollipops.

Form mini popcorn balls to the size desired. I like the mini size which is a ball that fits in the palm of my hand and is perfect to individually wrap for Halloween parties.

Place the popcorn balls on a baking sheet lined with parchment paper.

I had a package of candy eyeballs in the pantry so added one eyeball to each Pop for a Halloween touch, but the eyeball is optional!

Making Halloween Popcorn Balls Into Lollipops

By the time you are finished making 24 popcorn balls the popcorn balls will be ready for the lollipop sticks.

Insert the lollipop sticks.

Set the popcorn balls with the lollipop sticks.

I pop the lollipops in the refrigerator for a quick set, about 10-15 minutes.

You can leave the popcorn ball lollipops in longer, but warm to room temperature before serving.

These popcorn balls are fun! These are sticky! These are sweet and kids love them as an easy Halloween treat.

The mini Halloween Popcorn Ball Pops are also simple to package to make easy Halloween treats for school or parties.

After the Lollipops are set, inset each Pop in a clear cellophane bag and make use of your craft stash to use extra ribbon for the ties.

Easy as 1-2-3! I know there are 12 steps in the directions, but these Halloween treats are very fast to make especially if assembly line style is used.

I made 24 Pops in about 45 minutes including the time to set the popcorn balls. This Halloween I made a batch for the school fundraiser and the Halloween popcorn balls for sale were a hit and sold out quickly.

How To Make Orange Halloween Popcorn Lollipops

If you would like to add variety to your Popcorn Ball Pops skip the sprinkles. Simply add orange food coloring to the mixture for the Halloween season.

I did not have orange food coloring on hand and simply mixed the red and yellow food coloring with the popcorn ball mixture. Use multi color Lollipop sticks for a fun and slightly creepy Halloween food treat!

A second way to make orange popcorn balls adds a little more sweet to the mix with orange colored sugar. Actually any color of decorating sugar can be used.

Simply sprinkle the sugar on the completed lollipop before putting the lollipop in the refrigerator to set.

Fruit Infused Watermelon Ice Cubes

Easy and refreshing! This is a very flexible recipe and can be easily tweaked for your taste preference.

Course Drinks

Cuisine American

Keyword fruit infused watermelon ice cubes

Prep Time 15 minutes

Freeze 2 hours

Total Time 2 hours 15 minutes

Servings: 24 cubes

Ingredients:

1 1/2 cups watermelon

1/2 cup water

1 tablespoon honey

1 tablespoon lemon juice

Instructions:

Prepare your watermelon by cutting the watermelon into medium thick slices.

Remove the rind and seeds from the watermelon.

Seedless watermelon is highly recommended which will leave only a few white seeds to be removed.

Add all ingredients to a blender.

Puree.

Pour into ice cube trays. (even cuter are watermelon ice cube trays!) These make very cute watermelon shaped ice cubes which add a bit of fun and whimsy to the drinks.

Freeze.

Notes

If you are using a whole watermelon, I love this helpful watermelon slicing gadget to prep a whole watermelon.

A few hours are needed to freeze the watermelon puree into cubes.

Add the watermelon cubes to a glass of water or brighten up a glass of lemonade! Add a sprig of basil or mint to the glass or water for a festive and healthy drink.

Cauliflower Grits and Shrimp Recipe

Cauliflower Grits and Shrimp are easy enough for a busy weeknight, tasty enough for company and the perfect recipe for a low-carb, gluten-free diet!

Course: Main CourseCuisine: American Prep Time: 15 minutesCook Time: 15 minutesTotal Time: 30 minutes Servings: 4 servings Calories: 453kcal Author: Marjory Pilley

Ingredients:

4 cups cauliflower rice about 1 head of cauliflower

1 pound shrimp peeled and deveined

2 1/2 Tablespoons olive oil

1 Tablespoon Cajun spice

½ cup diced onion

2 garlic cloves minced

1 cup sharp cheddar cheese shredded

4 slices cooked and crumbled bacon or turkey bacon

¼ cup green onion chopped

Instructions:

Cut cauliflower florets from center stalk. Process florets in a food processor until they resemble "rice." Set aside.

Add shrimp, 2 Tablespoons of olive oil and Cajun spice to a bowl and stir to combine. Set aside.

Heat remaining oil in a frying pan over medium high heat.

Add onions and garlic and saute for about 3 minutes or until onions are soft.

Add cauliflower rice to pan and stir to combine.

Cover and cook for about 5 minutes.

Stir cheese into cauliflower rice.

Move rice to serving dish.

Add shrimp to skillet and cook over medium-high heat in a single layer for 3 minutes.

Stir and cook for about 3-4 minutes more or until shrimp is pink and cooked through.

Spoon shrimp over cauliflower rice and top with bacon and green onion.

Nutrition

Calories: 453kcal | Carbohydrates: 12g | Protein: 36g | Fat: 29g | Saturated Fat: 10g | Cholesterol: 329mg | Sodium: 1253mg | Potassium: 726mg | Fiber: 4g | Sugar: 4g | Vitamin A: 1205IU | Vitamin C: 84.9mg | Calcium: 419mg | Iron: 3.9mg

Low Oxalate Ham Broccoli Crustless Quiche

Light and airy low oxalate ham and broccoli crustless quiche the whole family can enjoy!

Course Main Course

Cuisine American

Prep Time 15 minutes

Cook Time 30 minutes

Total Time 45 minutes

Servings 4

Ingredients:

1 cup diced ham can use low salt ham

1 cup broccoli florets frozen or fresh

4 eggs

4 egg whites

1/4 cup water

1 cup low fat cottage cheese

White pepper to taste

Instructions:

Prepare a 9 " pie, baking dish or quiche dish with cooking spray.

Heat oven to 375 degrees.

Prepare your broccoli by pre cooking either in the microwave or on the stove top.

Dice the ham while the broccoli is cooking.

Using a large bowl, whisk the eggs, egg whites and water.

Now add the cottage cheese and whisk with intent! You want the cottage cheese to become fairly smooth and mix in with the egg mixture.

Pour into prepared dish. Place the broccoli and ham into the mixture.

Bake for 30 to 35 minutes. Check at the 30 minute mark.

As there is no crust, the top of the Ham And Broccoli Crustless Quiche will be slightly brown and the edges will be sightly brown also.

Notes

Not a cottage cheese fan? This is a great recipe to hide calcium friendly cottage cheese (especially for kids!)

Graham crackers and honey is a simple pairing of two low-oxalate ingredients, and an especially good option if the whole family is following a low-oxalate diet. You can make a big batch of honey and graham cracker sandwiches, and then keep them sealed in sandwich bags to carry during the day or pull from when you arrive home.

Serves: 4

Ingredients:

1 pound thick bacon cut into one-inch pieces

½ head iceberg or butter lettuce

10 cherry tomatoes

1 cup shredded cheddar cheese

Directions:

Cook bacon in a large skillet until evenly brown. Drain and set aside.

Cut cherry tomatoes into halves.

Sprinkle lettuce leaf with ¼ cup of cheddar cheese. Repeat for all tortillas.

Top each lettuce leaf with ¼ of bacon and cherry tomatoes.

Roll up wraps and cut in half.

LOW-OXALATE FRUIT SALAD

All you need are a few low-oxalate fruits cut into chunks, a small resealable bowl, and plastic fork for a portable, flavorful snack. Try these fruits with low levels of oxalate for your salad:

• Apples

• Bananas

• Pears

• Blueberries

You'll want to stay away from fruits with greater oxalate levels including raspberries, oranges, and kiwis.

BOXED RAISINS

Carry boxed raisins throughout your day so that you always have a low-oxalate boost of energy on hand. Raisins are a good source of carb, iron, potassium, calcium and protein as well as will satisfy your sweet tooth craving with only 130 calories per ¼ cup.

YOGURT CUPS

Most dairy products such as yogurt are low in oxalate and will also help you work towards a healthy calcium-oxalate ratio. Eat it plain or mix in low-oxalate fruits. Just be sure to avoid yogurts that come with nuts to mix-in, as these are often loaded with oxalate.

COCONUT FLOUR BANANA MUFFINS

This is another great bake that uses coconut flour as well as bananas, a low-oxalate fruit. This recipe is adapted from the Roasted Root.

Ingredients:

4 eggs, lightly beaten

4 ripe bananas, mashed

3 tablespoons maple syrup

2 teaspoons vanilla extract

½ cup coconut flour

½ teaspoon salt

1 teaspoon baking powder

½ teaspoon baking soda

Directions:

Preheat oven to 325 degrees Fahrenheit. Grease two muffin tins.

Combine eggs, banana, maple syrup and vanilla extract in a mixing bowl.

Stir coconut flour, salt, baking powder and baking soda in a mixing bowl.

Pour the dry mixture into the wet mixture and stir until combined. Batter should sit for five minutes before pouring into muffin tins.

Start checking that the dough is cooked at 20 minutes and keep baking until the muffins test clean.

PRETZELS

Eaten in moderation, pretzels will give you that crunch and salt you may be craving after giving up oxalate-packed snacks such as potato chips. Pretzels have a moderate level of oxalate and are easy to eat while you're working at your desk or on the move.

VANILLA PUDDING

You read right. Aside from being a dessert treat for kids, vanilla pudding cups are tasty, portable low-oxalate snacks. When eaten in moderation, these puddings can add some fun and nostalgia to your low-oxalate diet.

FETA DIP RECIPE
How To Make Feta Cheese Dip

INGREDIENTS:

6 ounce feta cheese (I use crumbled feta)

4 ounce of softened cream cheese

1/4 cup Greek or regular plain yogurt

1/8 cup good quality   Extra Virgin Olive Oil (EVOO) or Virgin Olive Oil

1 clove minced garlic

A smidge of lemon zest

Juice of 1/2 lemon

Garnish (optional) oregano or dill or parsley

DIRECTIONS:

Blend the feta cheese, cream cheese and yogurt to a whipped and smooth consistency. Use whichever tool your own – food processor, blender, electric mixer or hand mixer.

Add olive oil, garlic, lemon juice and a smidge of lemon zest.

Put dip into a decorative dip dish and add a spritz of olive oil and herb of your choice for a topping.

Crustless Asparagus Quiche

It's easy to fall in love with this Crustless Asparagus Quiche recipe. It's low-carb, gluten-free, presents beautifully and you can freeze it!

Course: BreakfastCuisine: French Prep Time: 10 minutesCook Time: 1 hourTotal Time: 1 hour 10 minutes Servings: 6 servings Calories: 182kcal Author: Marjory Pilley

Ingredients:

15-20 asparagus spears thin is best

5 eggs lightly beaten

1 cup milk (any type or combination will work. I use a mixture of skim milk and half and half.)

1/4 teaspoon salt

1/4 teaspoon white pepper

1/4 teaspoon thyme

1 cup Swiss cheese shredded

1/2 cup ham (optional) diced

Instructions:

Preheat oven to 350 degrees F.

Cut woody ends off of the asparagus spears.

Cut asparagus spears in half. Set top halves of spears aside and cut remaining halves in 1 inch segments.

Combine remaining ingredients, except for long pieces of asparagus spears and pie crust, if using, in a bowl.

Pour mixture into a 9 inch pan coated with cooking spray (or into the pie crust, if using.)

Using a fork, distribute ham, cheese and small asparagus pieces in pan.

Place long asparagus spears in a sunburst design. (See picture)

Bake quiche uncovered for 60-70 minutes or until an inserted knife comes out clean. The top should be lightly browned and the quiche will continue to set after removed from the oven.

Allow quiche to sit for 10-15 minutes before cutting.

Notes

Quiche can be frozen before or after cooking. Before cooking add all of the ingredients to a plastic bag that seals. Store in freezer. When ready to cook, defrost in the refrigerator, pour mixture into a pan and cook as directed. After cooking, wrap slices with plastic wrap and place in freezer. Slices can be re-heated in the microwave or oven.

Keep this recipe South Beach 1 compliant with low-fat milk and low-fat or fat-free cheese.

Nutrition

Calories: 182kcal | Carbohydrates: 4g | Protein: 14g | Fat: 11g | Saturated Fat: 5g | Cholesterol: 164mg | Sodium: 340mg | Potassium: 232mg | Sugar: 3g |

Vitamin A: 715IU | Vitamin C: 2.2mg | Calcium: 218mg | Iron: 1.6mg

EASY PALEO APPLE BUTTER

This easy Paleo apple butter is a delicious way to celebrate the fall.

15 min

Prep Time

5 hr

Cook Time

5 hr, 15

Total Time

Ingredients:

3 pounds of apples, your choice of variety

1/3 cup apple cider vinegar

cinnamon, nutmeg and cloves to taste

Instructions:

Peel and core the apples.

Put them in the slow cooker along with the apple cider vinegar.

Cook on high for three to four hours, stirring occasionally.

The apples should start to break down into chunks at this point.

Put them in the blender and blend until smooth.

Put them back into the slow cooker, add the spices, and cook (uncovered) for about half an hour more.

It is done when the apple butter starts to get thicker.

Refrigerate

Are you going on a low oxalate diet? These recipes are the perfect diet for you. Enjoy!

When it comes to an oxalate free diet, the key lies in playing about with the ingredients to find what works great for you. I hope that you enjoyed my low oxalate recipes and that you now have a clear idea as to what constitutes oxalate-free diets. Thank you!

www.ingramcontent.com/pod-product-compliance
Lightning Source LLC
Chambersburg PA
CBHW071549150726
48000CB00002B/994